CONQUERING VAGINISMUS

A Practical Guide to Pain-Less Sexual Health

Dr. Julianne

Copyright © 2023 by Dr. Julianne

2

Disclaimer

The information provided in this book is intended for educational and informational purposes only. It is not a substitute for professional medical advice, diagnosis, or treatment. Never disregard professional medical advice or delay in seeking it because of something you have read in this book. The author and publisher are not responsible for any actions or decisions you make based on the information provided in this book.

Results may vary and are not guaranteed. Individual responses to treatment and strategies discussed in this book may differ based on personal circumstances and medical history.

The author and publisher disclaim any liability for any adverse effects or consequences resulting from the use of information in this book.

Disclaimer

INTRODUCTION

Chapter 1

UNDERSTANDING VAGINISMUS

The Emotional Impact of Vaginismus

Physical Impact of Vaginismus

Chapter 2

SIGNS AND SYMPTOMS

Common Symptoms and Signs

Effect Of Vaginismus on Sexual Interaction

Impact on Relationship

Impact On Mental Health

Chapter 3

TYPES OF VAGINISMUS

Primary Vaginismus

Secondary Vaginismus

Chapter 4

CAUSES OF VAGINISMUS

Psychological Causes

Physical Causes

Misconceptions About Vaginismus

Chapter 5

TREATMENT OPTIONS FOR VAGINISMUS

Self-Help Techniques

Therapeutic Methods

Medical Procedures

Victorious Story Of A Woman With Vaginismus.

CONCLUSION

INTRODUCTION

It's not just you. I want you to know as you read this book that numerous others understand your battle, your suffering, and your will to overcome this pain. Your decision to read this book reveals a great deal about your bravery and willingness to take on the difficulties that vaginismus has presented to you.

There is a secret symphony of tales hidden in the quiet that frequently envelops the subject of vaginismus. Many people have battled quietly with this condition, feeling alone and misunderstood. However, you, my dear reader, have taken a different route. By seeking to read this book, you're saying, "I am ready to seek help, to understand, and to heal."

It's challenging enough to talk about something as delicate as vaginismus. The layers of shame and embarrassment that society has piled on top of us must be removed. But it's in these discussions that we find comfort and vigor. It is impossible to overstate the importance of discussing vaginism openly. It's about breaking free from the bonds of silence and allowing your voice to be heard alongside the countless others who have gone through or are going through the same struggle.

The simple yet profound goal of this book is to accompany you on this journey by acting as your guide and source of hope. It serves as a testament to the strength of knowledge, empathy, and practical options.

We will explore the causes, emotional toll, and potential treatments of vaginismus as we unravel the complexities of the condition through these pages. We will give you advice based on our combined knowledge of medicine and personal experience because we think both are essential to your recovery.

However, this book offers more than just facts. It is a proclamation that you are entitled to a life free of vaginismus. It's a confirmation that your suffering is real, that you are understood, and that pursuing your desires for intimacy is worthwhile. It's a rallying cry to fight the stigma that has kept so many people hidden in the dark.

Therefore, keep in mind that you are not on this journey alone while you read the pages that follow. You are a warrior who rejects the vaginismus' attempt to define you. You are moving closer to taking back control of your body, your pleasure, and your life with every word you read and piece of advice you ingest.

8

Chapter 1

UNDERSTANDING VAGINISMUS

Vaginismus is the medical term for the uncontrollable tightening of the muscles surrounding the vaginal entrance, which makes penetration unpleasant, uncomfortable, and even impossible. Lots of instances, including attempted sex, gynecological check-ups, or even just the idea of penetration, can cause this tightness.

Imagine an unconscious reaction that causes the muscles surrounding the vagina to contract in anticipation of a threat. Vaginismus—a condition where the body's instincts react to intimacy with anxiety and resistance.

It may be confusing or even disappointing to hear this statement, but it's important to understand that vaginismus isn't a choice. It's not a sign of resistance or lack of interest. It's a complicated combination of psychological, emotional, and physical components that come together to produce a problem that seems insurmountable.

Vaginismus doesn't affect or adhere to your ability to be aroused and enjoy other forms of sexual activity.

You might be shocked to realize the extent to which vaginismus is common, considering how unheard of it is. Millions of women are said to be afflicted by this condition worldwide. But because of the silence that surrounds it, many women find themselves alone and think they are the only ones going through this experience.

The Emotional Impact of Vaginismus

Imagine living a life where something as normal as intimacy becomes a cause of anxiety and annoyance. This is a reality for many who live with vaginismus, it's not simply their imagination. The emotional effects can be profound. From perplexity and embarrassment to fury and despair, it's a rollercoaster of emotions.

Vaginismus frequently shows up unannounced, leaving you confused and ashamed. The sense of inadequacy and the belief that your body is fundamentally failing you are the root of the embarrassment Those who are affected frequently distance themselves from their spouses out of a sense of rejection and judgment.

Strained Relationship: Intimacy which is the foundation of relationships can turn into a battlefield. Your husband can find it difficult to comprehend the condition, unintentionally causing a rift. It may lead you to feel extremely guilty about not living up to your husband's expectations.

Isolation and Misunderstanding: Regardless of their sincere efforts, friends and family members may fail to understand the complex nature of vaginismus. This lack of understanding can lead to a sense of isolation, as you might feel unable to confide in those nearest to you. The emotional pain of vaginismus can be as difficult as the physical pain.

Physical Impact of Vaginismus

Vaginismus exacts a physical price that cannot be disregarded in addition to the emotional cost. By upsetting the body's natural harmony, it alters what ought to be enjoyable into a painful experience.

The Pain Barrier:

Penetration is difficult, if not impossible, due to the involuntary contractions that take place during vaginismus. This pain perpetuates a cycle of anxiety and discomfort by serving as a persistent reminder of the body's resistance. This may eventually cause the affected area to become hypersensitive to touch.

Sexual Dysfunction:

Vaginismus can cause sexual dysfunction due to its physical restrictions. This can include a variety of difficulties, such as the inability to arouse or have orgasms. The emotional toll can be made worse by the frustration and disappointment that come along with these occurrences.

Body Image and Confidence:

There is a strong link between body image and confidence. Vaginismus can lower self-esteem, making people feel unattractive and out of control over their bodies. This could create an endless circle where the more one's self-esteem declines, the more severe the physical symptoms become.

Met Sarah....................

Sarah says vaginismus had a huge impact on her life, resulting in broken relationships, damaged self-worth, isolation, and a lot of money spent.

"I previously thought about seeing a sex therapist but decided against it because of the expensive consultations and my discomfort dealing with a male therapist. I went to a renowned gynecologist, who gave me a terrible penetrative checkup with a speculum before telling me to stop taking things so seriously. After that, I went to visit family in another country and used the time to schedule sessions with a sexological bodyworker. Her method was extremely kind, and the hands-on sessions were incredibly helpful for me in letting go of my guilt, feeling more at ease in my nervous system, and removing some layers of trauma."

We must understand that vaginismus is not an abstract concept – it's a deeply personal struggle that affects relationships, self-worth, and daily life. It's a testament to the fortitude of the human spirit, a journey that entails learning and ultimately healing.

Chapter 2

SIGNS AND SYMPTOMS

Vaginismus is an underlying condition that manifests both physically and mentally in a variety of ways. Recognizing the signs and symptoms is the first step to understanding your experience and getting the appropriate assistance. In this chapter, we'll discuss the typical vaginismus symptoms and consider how they could affect social interactions, sexual behavior, and mental health.

Common Symptoms and Signs

1. Muscles That Contract Involuntarily

The distinguishing characteristic of vaginismus is the involuntary contractions of the muscles surrounding the vaginal entrance, which renders penetration uncomfortable or possibly impossible. This might take place during intercourse, pelvic examinations, or tampon use.

2. Pain During Penetration

Trying to enter the vagina can be excruciating for women with vaginismus. The pain can range from mild to excruciating, and it is commonly described as a burning or stinging feeling.

3. Fear & worry

Just the idea of suffering can cause intense dread and worry. People who are worried about getting wounded during penetration may enter a vicious cycle in which their anxiety causes them to tense their muscles.

4. Avoidance Behavior

People with vaginismus may completely avoid sexual activity due to the discomfort and anxiety brought on by penetration. This avoidance can make relationships difficult and prevent emotional closeness.

5. Reduced Sexual Desire

The pain and anxiety of penetration might cause a reduction in sexual desire. The overall enjoyment of sexual activities can be impacted by one's negative connections with intimacy.

6. Feeling "Blocked" or "Unnatural"

Some women with vaginismus say that their husbands experience a physical block or barrier that makes penetration feel impossible for them. Feelings of frustration and inadequacy may result from this.

Effect Of Vaginismus on Sexual Interaction

Vaginismus has a significant negative effect on sexual relationships, making what ought to be a delightful and intimate experience, one that is rife with discomfort and worry. A cycle of anxiety and avoidance results from the uncontrollable muscle contractions that make penetration painful or impossible. The fear of pain can also lessen desire and lubrication, which makes penetration more challenging.

Impact on Relationship

Vaginismus affects relationships on many different levels, going beyond just physical discomfort. As spouses struggle to cope with the emotional toll of the condition, communication may become difficult. The avoidance behaviors that result from a fear of intimacy and pain can destroy romantic chemistry and emotional closeness. The frustration and solitude experienced by women with vaginismus may be unintentionally increased by partners who find it difficult to comprehend the illness.

Impact On Mental Health

Both partners' mental health may suffer as a result of vaginismus's emotional toll. Shame, inadequacy, and self-doubt are frequent feelings. Negative self-image and low self-esteem might result from being unable to have the desired sexual experiences. The condition's frustration and displeasure can exacerbate anxiety and despair, which can have a general negative influence that impacts the overall quality of life.

Chapter 3

TYPES OF VAGINISMUS

Vaginismus encompasses different forms that manifest with unique characteristics and triggers. Understanding these two categories—primary and secondary—can help you better comprehend your personal experiences as well as discover the underlying causes and choose the best method of treatment.

Primary Vaginismus

Consider yourself at the front of a door that, despite your best efforts to open, will not budge. This is the basis of primary vaginismus. It is characterized by an uncontrollable tightening of the pelvic muscles, making penetration uncomfortable and impossible from the very beginning, whether it be with a tampon, a finger, or a partner.

Causes

Primary vaginismus frequently results from psychological issues including anxiety, pain phobia, or bad connections with sex.

The emergence of primary vaginismus may be influenced by traumatic events, conservative parenting, or cultural beliefs.

In other instances, it may also be related to a lack of sexual education where the body's natural response to penetration is one of defense.

25-year-old Claire has been in an amazing relationship for a while. However, despite her partner's compassion and patience, every attempt at sexual activity results in a reflexive tightening of her vaginal muscles, which causes excruciating pain. Sarah has primary vaginismus as a result of her body's instinctive reaction and her dread of pain.

In her fight against vaginismus, she discovered that she had mentally hidden something within her subconscious that made her think of sex as something she doesn't want, so her body's reaction is to close up as a means of defense. After one and a half years of marriage without consummation, she finally broke through the issue of vaginismus after breaking through the thoughts in her subconscious.

Secondary Vaginismus

Now picture a door that was open at one time but has since been gradually closed. This is secondary vaginismus. In contrast to primary vaginismus, it appears when a woman has previously been able to engage in sexual activity without pain or difficulty.

Causes

- Inflammatory diseases of the pelvis or vaginal infections are examples of physical conditions.
- Psychological elements like anxiety or trauma, or particular drugs.
- Sexual or physical abuse
- Medical operations, including childbirth and surgery.

You can work toward specific remedies if you are aware of whether your experience is consistent with primary or secondary vaginismus. Keep in mind that you are not on this journey alone. Many people have had the same difficulties and have discovered solutions.

Chapter 4

CAUSES OF VAGINISMUS

Psychological Causes

1. Fear and Anxiety

Fear can be a powerful trigger for vaginismus. Negative attachment to sex, pain, or traumatic experiences can lead to an unconscious fear of penetration. The body's natural response to this fear is to tighten the vaginal muscles, creating a cycle of pain and anxiety.

2. Past Trauma

Sexual or non-sexual traumas in a person's past can profoundly influence their experience of vaginismus. These traumas might be buried in the subconscious, causing the body to react defensively during attempts at penetration.

3. Cultural and Religious Factors

Upbringing in conservative cultures or religious backgrounds that stigmatize or suppress discussions about sex can contribute to vaginismus. Lack of sexual education and guilt associated with sexual activities can intensify anxiety and muscle tension.

4. Relationship Dynamics

Relationship issues, lack of emotional intimacy, or communication problems with a partner can contribute to vaginismus. Emotional well-being and a sense of safety are closely intertwined with sexual experiences.

Physical Causes

1. Infections and Medical Conditions

Infections of the genital area, like yeast infections or urinary tract infections, can cause discomfort and pain during penetration, triggering vaginismus. Certain medical conditions like endometriosis, pelvic inflammatory disease, or even vulvodynia can contribute to muscle tension.

2. Hormonal Changes

Various fluctuations in hormone levels, often experienced during pregnancy, breastfeeding, or menopause, can lead to vaginal dryness and discomfort. This physical discomfort can subsequently trigger vaginismus.

3. Surgical Procedures

Surgeries in the pelvic region, such as hysterectomy or episiotomy, can leave scar tissue that leads to muscle spasms and pain during penetration, contributing to vaginismus.

4. Medications

Some medications can result in dryness or changes in vaginal tissue, causing discomfort and pain during intercourse. The resulting discomfort can perpetuate the cycle of vaginismus.

Misconceptions About Vaginismus

Myth 1: You're Not Trying Hard Enough

Vaginismus does not require effort or willpower. Since there is no conscious way to stop involuntary muscular contractions, it is a real medical problem that needs to be understood and treated.

Myth 2: You're alone because it's rare

Vaginismus is more widespread than you might imagine, but because of shame, many people remain silent about their suffering. There is a network of people who support one another and who have been on the same road as you, so you are not alone.

Myth 3: Only women who haven't had sex are affected.

Regardless of their past sexual behavior, anyone can experience vaginismus. It may start after years of pain-free intimacy owing to illnesses, trauma, or other circumstances.

Myth 4: It's Just Nerves

Although worry and uneasiness might be a factor, vaginismus is a nuanced condition with many underlying causes that go beyond simple anxiety.

Myth 5: Vaginismus won't require treatment and will go away

If you've always found sex to be unpleasant, staying the same won't likely make things better. It can worsen vaginismus and enhance your body's relationship between pain and penetrative sex. Simply "trying to relax" will not have an impact because a relaxation response cannot be forced.

Myth 6: Since it cannot be treated, you should give up

There is no way that this myth is true. A variety of methods, including physical therapy, counseling, education, and open communication with your spouse, can be used to treat vaginismus successfully.

Chapter 5

TREATMENT OPTIONS FOR VAGINISMUS

Self-Help Techniques

It is essential to empower yourself to take an active role in your recovery process. Add these self-help practices to your routine each day:

1. Educational Exploration:

Understanding is a useful tool. Start by becoming knowledgeable about your own body's mechanics and demystifying the penetration process. Fears and concerns may be lessened as a result.

2. Exercises for the Pelvis:

The management of vaginismus can benefit considerably by strengthening the pelvic floor muscles. Kegel exercises and yoga-inspired poses that emphasize calmness and control can help with better muscle coordination.

3. Breathing Exercises

Your nervous system can be calmed and your muscles can loosen up with deep, controlled breathing, allowing you to approach intimacy with ease.

4. Desensitization

Your body can gradually develop more accustomed to intimacy by exposing you to various types of touch and sensations over time.

5. Partner Participation

Vaginismus affects the spouse as well as the individual. Including your partner in your journey helps promote tolerance, openness, and understanding. Their assistance can serve as a potent stimulant for development.

Therapeutic Methods

Professional advice is a guiding light for you. Consult therapists who have training in sexual health, trauma, or anxiety. While trauma therapists can address underlying emotional scars, sex therapists can lead you through customized tactics.

1. Cognitive-Behavioral Therapy (CBT)

Attending therapy can assist you in recognizing and reframing unfavorable thought patterns and intercourse-related fears. CBT can offer coping mechanisms and management techniques for managing triggers successfully.

2. Sex Therapy

To address the psychological and physical components of vaginismus, work with a certified sex therapist. They can lead you through ways to improve intimacy, sensory exploration, and communication activities.

3. Counseling for couples

Vaginismus can make relationships difficult. Couples counseling helps partners communicate openly and with empathy and understanding, which helps to create a supportive environment for tackling the disease together.

Medical Procedures

Lubricants, moisturizers, and topical numbing agents are some topical treatments that might assist in reducing discomfort during penetration. Before using any items, check with a healthcare practitioner to be sure they are secure and appropriate for you.

1. Dilators

Graduated dilators can gently stretch and train the vaginal muscles to relax, reducing the instinctive response of contraction. Smaller dilators are used first, then larger ones.

2. Botox injections

In some situations, it may be possible to temporarily relax the muscles around the vagina to facilitate painless entry. Usually, this is carried out with the assistance of a medical expert.

3. Medication

Certain drugs, such as muscle relaxants or low-dose anxiety medications, may be recommended to relieve the mental and emotional stress related to vaginismus. But they must be used following a medical practitioner's description.

Victorious Story Of A Woman With Vaginismus.

Working with women with vaginismus for almost 7 years has taught us how isolating and alone this condition can make one feel. Women struggle with this secret and it takes tremendous courage to reach out and seek treatment.

We want to share a recent success story of a woman who overcame vaginismus by facing her worries. Her story is motivational, and hopefully, it will inspire other women who are suffering in silence to get assistance.

"A few months ago, if you had asked me to describe my medical path or treatment for Vaginismus, I definitely would have broken down in tears just by expressing how helpless I felt. I was certain that having sex would not be possible for me.

Vaginismus is a monster that isolates. That's pretty much the best way I can put it. It leaves you feeling misunderstood by everyone, shattered and unfixable, powerless despite valiant efforts, and betrayed by your own body. You feel upset because, despite being a highly reasonable person in every other scenario, you just can't get your body to listen to you or grasp what is happening.

I was never able to use a tampon, never had a gynecological exam, and was never allowed to engage in sexual activity as a child. I was aware that the tampon issue was peculiar, but I never gave it much thought.

I visited my gynecologist during my time in college to have a regular exam that I had never had before. Because of my anxiety, I can still recall feeling my body starting to sweat profusely. My doctor told me to return when I was sexually active and that she wouldn't "violate" me today because I hadn't been able to use tampons or have sex. Due to my resolve to wait until marriage, I wasn't sexually active when I became engaged, but I went to a new doctor to receive birth control for when I got married. I repeated my inability to use a tampon, lack of exam experience, and lack of sex history.

This physician advised me to return a few months after getting married when I was accustomed to having things in there, to discuss the issue further.

Fast-forward to my honeymoon. We tried several times, but sex just wasn't working for us. My husband would describe it as feeling like he was striking a brick wall. He had no chance of entering. It was simply painful for me. My husband was very thoughtful, but we were both dissatisfied. We decided to just give it time when we got home, blaming it on the fact that it was new to me.

We decided to start couples therapy after about six months of trying without success. Our counselor informed us a few months later that she suspected it was vaginismus and advised us to research it. were relieved to have a potential solution, so that evening we searched it up at home and discovered a vaginismus expert who sold dilators and instructional books. In a hurry to find a solution, we bought them.

They spent months in our room after they came, doing nothing. I was already hesitant to attempt to use the dilators after taking them out of their packaging. When I did try to insert the tiniest dilator, approximately the size of a pinky, it seemed like I was hitting a wall.

I decided to try seeing a midwife after a few more months of hiding out alone in my turmoil. She decided that it would be better if I underwent an examination under anesthesia once I was there and it became evident that I could not undergo an examination. I had suggested that it may be vaginismus, but she concluded that my hymen was the problem. That sent me on a path of MRIs, doctors, and unsuccessful surgery.

After everything had been tried and tested, the gynecologist recommended that I see a physical therapist to work on the pelvic floor muscles (the same muscles associated with vaginismus), which included using a dilator.

Exhausted, defeated, and hopeless my sweet cousin sent an email of a video of a girl who used [a medication] to cure Vaginismus. Instantly I started researching possible ways, by reading books and meeting specialized therapist

I was in tears when I began reading reviews. I couldn't believe that other women were going through the same thing as me and that they were surviving.

I had a meeting with a consultant who was truly a blessing. The women I spoke with gave me hope and reassuring encouragement that there are a lot of other women who deal with this. I immediately began the process to complete the treatment. I received a call from the consultant, who I firmly believe to be an angel, a few weeks later. She was kind, understanding, and knowledgeable.

She was able to truly explain medically what was wrong after hearing from everyone up to this point that I should just relax, that it would happen, or that I was worrying about it too much. She was the complete opposite of the treatment I had received thus far from doctors and gynecologists. She explained to me that while the treatment is beneficial, the PT done with the dilators following the procedure is just as crucial, if not more so. I immediately conveyed my worry about how I had previously been unable to utilize dilators and how I was certain I would fail.

She boosted my confidence and gave me encouragement, which helped me to feel even better about my choice to pursue this. A little over a month later, I made the trip to have the procedure done.

When I eventually saw the consultant in person, she once more went over the entire process with me. She explained to me that she would use the dilator on me for almost an hour right after the procedure. I was anxious once more, but I was willing to try anything. When I went in for the process, I had the biggest dilator inside of me when I woke up from the anesthetic. I couldn't believe there was something inside of me and it didn't hurt. I was able to use the biggest dilator when she arrived. I found it really hard to believe. We then replaced it with a medium dilator, which I took with me home and slept in all night.

I was certain, when I returned to my hotel, that I couldn't do the dilators on my own and that I was simply acting courageous in front of the doctors. I was anxious about having to re-insert the dilator when I went to the restroom. But there was no discomfort when I inserted the dilator again! The next day, when I went for my follow-up visit, she showed me how to use the dilators and I was able to go back up to the biggest one. All I felt was joy. For the first time, I no longer felt confined to my ruined body.

After returning home, I kept using my dilators. As directed, I utilized them for 30 minutes each day. They actually started to soothe me in a way, which shocked me greatly. I got along well with them! I was extremely joyful and certain after it! Weekly check-ins with the consultant to see how I was doing and if I needed anything. I was able to use a tampon that month when my period started. I was excited to discuss it with her even though my husband and I still hadn't had any luck with sex.

She was able to examine me (never done before!) and gave me several options for how to continue with my physical therapy in order to be successful. My husband and I had our first sexual intercourse a week later! I never anticipated living to see the day. Since we've been together for over two and a half years, it's safe to say that neither of us had any thoughts that our intimacy would ever return to normal in our marriage".

CONCLUSION

As you end this chapter, remember that vaginismus is not who you are; rather, it is a chapter in your story, one that you can change. The path to recovery may be rocky and paved with obstacles, but it is a path paved with possibilities that lead to freedom and hope.

Accept this path wholeheartedly. Accept your capacity for growth and development, your ability to enjoy yourself, and the grace of your tenacity. You're getting closer to the life you deserve with each step you take—a life filled with intimacy confidence, and the profound delight of taking back control of your body and your pleasure.

May this book serve as a continual reminder that you already possess the power to triumph, the bravery to accept change, and the wisdom to go with grace on this road. Your narrative is one of success, and your path to recovery is evidence of the amazing power you possess.